Young Carers
in Their Own Words

Edited by Andrew Bibby and Saul Becker

CALOUSTE GULBENKIAN FOUNDATION, LONDON

Published by the
Calouste Gulbenkian Foundation
United Kingdom Branch
98 Portland Place
London W1N 4ET
Tel: 020 7636 5313

ISBN 0 903319 93 4

British Library Cataloguing-in-Publication Data
A catalogue record for this book is available from
the British Library

Designed by Andrew Shoolbred
Printed by Expression Printers Ltd, IP23 8HH

Distributed by Turnaround Publisher Services Ltd,
Unit 3, Olympia Trading Estate, Coburg Road, Wood Green,
London N22 6TZ.
Tel: 020 8829 3000, Fax: 020 8881 5088,
E-mail: orders@turnaround-uk.com

Contents

Foreword by Ben Whitaker   6

Introduction   7

Chapter 1: The Position of Young Carers Today   11

Chapter 2: Young Carers and Public Policy   25

Young Carers in Their Own Words   43

Good Practice Checklists   71

References and Further Reading   79

Foreword

One of the most intractable challenges faced by grant-giving foun-
dations is that those people who apply to them for funding are not
necessarily the most meritorious or in need. Young carers – among the
most hidden of all groups in our society – are probably the least likely
of any to know about grant-giving bodies, let alone apply to one. In
addition they are unfortunately too often inhibited from asking for
help from adults or those in authority because of the fear that if they
do so their ill or disabled parent would be taken away and they themselves put into care.

Yet few young people more genuinely merit our admiration and
support. Often these children have surrendered much of their childhood to their family responsibilities: too tired to cope at school, too
embarrassed to invite friends home. When is one of them ever able to
lobby their MP or councillor, or write to the media? This is why
Andrew Bibby and Saul Becker's book, with the voices of the young
carers themselves, should be read by all the rest of us who have been
lucky enough not to have been asked to carry such responsibilities –
and then we should not delay acting to do what we can to help them
and their families.

Ben Whitaker

Introduction

This book presents written accounts by children and young people of what it is like to be a carer. As individuals they differ in many respects: where they live, who they live with, their family backgrounds and ethnic origins, and their age (the youngest contributor is nine, the oldest 18) but what they have in common – and what distinguishes them from others of their own generation – is that they are all taking on significant caring responsibilities for one or more members of their family with a disability or illness.

The government's National Strategy for Carers, published in 1999, recognises the existence of such 'young carers' and makes a number of recommendations for action, based on an understanding that young carers have their particular needs and can legitimately make certain demands of the rest of society. One of their needs, according to the National Strategy for Carers, is for there to be recognition of the role they perform. This is, in a sense, the starting point for this book. It is an attempt to allow young carers to speak directly of their lives and their experiences.

Most people consider that it is appropriate to ask their children, as they grow older, to play an increasing part in the collective work of running the family household: day-to-day tasks like washing up, tidying the house, or keeping an eye on younger siblings. The work which young carers do, however, is of a significantly different order from this. *The Blackwell Encyclopaedia of Social Work* defines young carers as those people under 18 who 'carry out, often on a regular basis, significant or substantial caring tasks, and assume a level of responsibility which would usually be associated with an adult'. Typically they will be looking after one of their parents who is disabled, has a chronic illness or is suffering from mental health problems. Some young carers care for a grandparent, a brother or sister, or other relative. Some care for more than one person.

Not much more than ten years ago, there was almost no public recognition that some children and young people were taking on these roles. Jill Pitkeathley (now Baroness Pitkeathley) has recalled how in the mid-1980s she and others in Carers National Association faced 'incredulity' when they tried to point out that many young children were carrying out major caring responsibilities. No one really believed that young carers existed.

Since then the situation has changed. Gradually, through the efforts of a small number of researchers and campaigners, public attention has been focused on the issue. The term 'young carers' has gained increasing currency in academic, social care and social policy circles, and has also become one which the children and young people themselves are likely to recognise and use. Labels like this can be useful if they help validate an experience which might otherwise remain inchoate and unarticulated.

The decision to publish this collection of experiences by children who are carers was taken by Ben Whitaker, who recently retired as Director of the Calouste Gulbenkian Foundation. For several years the Foundation has helped fund research projects and initiatives designed to draw attention to the situation of young carers. The work of collecting and editing the contributions has been undertaken jointly by Andrew Bibby, an independent writer and journalist, and by Saul Becker, Director of the Young Carers Research Group at Loughborough University. One of us was approaching the issue of young carers for the first time in compiling this book, the other has been closely identified with the subject for the past decade. The introduction and chapters have been written by Andrew Bibby, the good practice checklists (pages 71–8) were supplied by Saul Becker; however, the book itself is a joint endeavour.

The children and young people whose views are recorded here were reached primarily through the network of locally based young carers projects. At the start of the 1990s, there were only two local projects in Britain which aimed to support the work of young carers. Now there are well over 100 such groups. We contacted each group and asked them to let young carers in their area know about the work we were undertaking. We produced a short flyer, which asked: 'What's good and bad about your life? We are looking for articles, stories, poems etc., from young people and children who are caring for other members of their family, reflecting their experiences.' About 160 contributions were initially received, from which we made the current selection. We were looking for contributions which gave readers an insight into the lives of young carers. We omitted some interesting and powerful writing on the grounds that it dealt essentially with the experiences of young people as young people – rather than specifically with those aspects of their lives which related to their work as young carers.

When we discussed the initial selection we had made we were conscious, however, that there were gaps. Caring can involve many things, including coping with physical and emotional aspects of life which all of us – adult and child alike – tend not to talk about, or at least not to people we do not know very well. If this collection was to reflect as comprehensively as possible the different facets of being a young carer (including the painful aspects of coping with very unwell people), this problem had to be addressed. We therefore decided to extend the collection by including extracts taken from a series of structured conversations ('conversations with a purpose') held with older young carers in 1999 by Chris Dearden of the Young Carers Research Group. We are very grateful to Chris, and to the Joseph Rowntree Foundation (which funded the research), and to the young carers themselves, for allowing us to use these extracts, which would otherwise have remained unpublished in these longer versions.

The conversations were taped and fully transcribed, and, as with the written contributions, editorial intervention has been kept to the minimum. Sometimes, however, the text removes some hesitations and pauses and occasionally runs together the answers to different questions. The interview extracts are identified by a grey border.

The collection clearly reveals the issues and concerns which young carers face, not least in their relations with adults in positions of professional responsibility. The aim of Chapter 1 is to help provide a context for these writings. As will be seen, a once-ignored social issue has in ten years produced a considerable bank of research findings, new policies and initiatives.

Chapter 2 goes on to consider issues of public policy. There is now at least some recognition of young carers in government pronouncements and a degree of understanding of the issue among (some) health and social care professionals. However, considerable numbers of children and young people are still coping with a caring role without the level of support or understanding which a civilised society should be able to offer.

Chapter 1

The Position of Young Carers Today

Who are the young carers?

A surprisingly large number of children live in households where at least one member of the family is hampered in their daily life by chronic physical or mental health problems or by disability. Almost three million (just under a quarter of all children in Britain) find themselves living in these sorts of households.

Not all of these children, of course, take on a caring role. The Department of Health has defined young carers as those people under 18 who provide 'a substantial amount of care on a regular basis', though government guidelines also make it clear that some young people with less regular or substantial caring commitments may still face the kinds of difficulties and disadvantages associated with being a young carer.

It is not necessarily easy for the outside world to know when caring is taking place within the family home. The Office for National Statistics (ONS) states that up to 51,000 children can be classified as young carers. Some researchers suggest that this figure is an underestimate, and that there are many young carers who carry on their lives completely hidden from officialdom.

It is also worth noting – even assuming that the ONS figure of 51,000 is approximately right – that many of these are not in touch with social workers or other professionals. Only about 5,000 young carers are actively known to the network of workers in young carers groups and projects and a much smaller number of these have had formal assessments of their needs carried out, the procedure by which carers' requirements for assistance can be identified. The right to ask for an assessment was given to carers (including young carers) in the 1995 Carers (Recognition and Services) Act.

The largest survey of young carers in Britain was undertaken in 1997 by the Young Carers Research Group (YCRG), with the findings published a year later in the book *Young Carers in the UK*. This research project surveyed just over 2,300 children and young people, the vast majority of whom were of school age (i.e. under 16).

Their findings were revealing. Over half (54%) of these young carers lived in lone-parent families, and in these cases the child or young person was typically looking after their ill or disabled parent (more often than not, the mother). The survey also revealed that 12% were caring for more than one person.

It is possible that the immediate picture conjured up by the term 'young carer' is that of a teenage girl helping to care for her mother, who is, say, disabled and a wheelchair user. But this is not necessarily a typical picture. Firstly, a considerable number of children and young people are caring for someone who is suffering from mental, rather than physical, ill health. This can include manic depression, schizophrenia, alcohol misuse or drug dependency.

Secondly, young carers may be younger (perhaps significantly younger) than many people might imagine: the YCRG found that the average age of the young carers surveyed was 12 and their past research work has found children undertaking caring at age five or even younger.

Finally, while it seems that girls are more likely than boys to be taking on the caring role, the gender difference is not particularly striking: 43% of the young carers surveyed in 1997 were boys.

What sort of care do these young carers provide? Researchers have tended to categorise the work undertaken in a number of ways, distinguishing between domestic, personal and emotional tasks. The first category would include such things as cooking meals, cleaning the house, washing and ironing clothes. Personal care ranges from simply ensuring that the person being cared for has their medication at the right time to very intimate tasks, such as washing, showering or toileting.

The 1997 YCRG survey went further in terms of categorising young carers' tasks. It found that 72% undertook domestic work, and 57% engaged in 'general' care (such as giving medication or helping with mobility). Forty-three per cent offered emotional support, particularly where a young carer was looking after someone with a mental health problem. Twenty-nine per cent undertook 'other' caring work, including money management, dealing with professionals, and translating for adults whose first language was not English, while a small number of young carers were *also* undertaking childcare for (healthy) younger siblings.

A surprisingly high number of children and young people were undertaking what the researchers described as intimate personal care: 449 of the 2,303 children and young people surveyed (21%) were in this category. This finding echoed a smaller survey undertaken by the YCRG two years earlier, where the equivalent percentage was 23%.

It is clear that there is a continuum of care being provided, from basic domestic tasks to very intimate care. It is also true that, for any individual child or young person, the burden of caring can shift along this continuum, if for example the person they are caring for becomes more seriously ill (or, conversely, if they are provided with additional professional help). The government's National Strategy for Carers puts it like this:

> There may be only a narrow dividing line between 'helping around the house' which many children do, and providing personal care for a relative. But, in the worst cases, young carers can be harmed by the responsibilities and expectations placed upon them. Many children will provide help and support in these situations: some will take on, perhaps gradually, significant responsibilities...

Public attitudes to young carers

Now that the evidence has come to light, how do we as a society respond to the issue of young carers? The presence of young carers poses something of a challenge to adult society: after all, we tend to have a set idea of what makes up a 'proper' childhood and of what constitutes the child's appropriate role and place in an adult-run world. Caring for disabled or seriously ill adults is not an activity which sits comfortably within this paradigm of childhood.

As David Deacon, a lecturer in media studies at Loughborough University, has pointed out, the response can be unsatisfactorily simplistic. Deacon has explored the attitude of the media to the young carers issue and has identified two dominant tendencies. The first he describes as the 'little angel' approach, typified by an article in the *London Evening Standard* in 1994 which carried the headline 'Two angels named Charlie are Britain's most caring children'. As Deacon says, this involves 'the eulogising of children who display unexpected levels of courage, selflessness and maturity in the face of considerable adversity'.

The other media approach is described by Deacon as portraying the young carer as 'the little victim'. He quotes a number of headlines to illustrate this, including one from *The Independent* in 1994 ('Children Aged 3 "Forced to Care for Disabled"') and another from *The Guardian* in the same year ('Unaided, Unpaid, Unsung'). He adds: 'In a high proportion of headlines and lead paragraphs, caring is recurrently referred to as a "burden" that falls on "young shoulders".'

It is clear that both the 'little angel' and the 'little victim' angles are inadequate, although it is also easy to see why they make for good newspaper copy and TV programming. To be fair, the media have played a role in bringing the young carer issue out from academic and professional circles to a wider audience (the first major TV programme on the subject was in fact broadcast by the BBC as long ago as 1985).

There is another reason, however, why even sophisticated versions of the 'little angel' or 'little victim' approach are inadequate, and that is that they marginalise the person who is receiving support from the young carer. As David Deacon puts it: 'In most press reports these people have a shadowy presence. They are hardly ever quoted directly, and when biographical details are provided they invariably concentrate on the nature or extent of their illness or disability…' Instead there is a lack of interest in the perspectives of recipients of care, '… and ready characterisation of the caring relationship as one of "dependency"…'

This is exactly the approach to disability which has been so robustly criticised in recent years by disability rights campaigners, particularly by people with disabilities who are determined not to be trapped by the imposed role of victim-dependant. The disability rights movement has challenged the traditional 'medical' approach to disability, which has tended to view disability as a deviation from an implied norm and which has indirectly done much to disempower people with disabilities.

In contrast, the disability rights critique which has been developed recently argues that, if there is a disability 'problem', it is not with disabled people themselves but rather with a society which is organised in such a way that people with disabilities are prevented from playing a full part. One could say, for example, that the problem is not the wheelchair but the absence of buildings where wheelchairs can be used.

This point will be considered in more detail in the following chapter, but it should be stressed here that one cannot and should not consider the interests and rights of young carers without at the same time looking at the interests and rights of the people being cared for. Without this perspective, any approach to the issue of young carers at best risks being one-sided, while at worst it could reinforce unacceptable stereotypes of disability.

Another important point is that the experience of being a young carer is not always entirely negative. There are positive aspects, too. In their recently published report *Growing Up Caring* (a study of 60 older young carers, aged 16–25) Chris Dearden and Saul Becker make the following observation:

> Many of the young people viewed the maturity, responsibility, independence and life skills they had acquired in a positive light. They could see that these would be useful to them throughout life and felt better prepared for adulthood than many of their peers. About a quarter of all the respondents mentioned these qualities as being the best part of helping to care for and support a parent who was ill or disabled.
>
> Other comments on the positive nature of caring were gaining an understanding about illness and disability and having a caring attitude towards others. Seven respondents specifically mentioned the closeness of their relationships with their parents.

Nevertheless, there are certainly negative aspects. As the authors of *Growing Up Caring* report: 'The negative impacts included stress and depression, restricted social, educational and career opportunities, and less time for oneself.' These can have serious implications for children's psycho-social development and their transition to adulthood.

The rest of this chapter will look at some of the major issues raised by the caring work undertaken by children and young people. Some of the negative impacts are, of course, likely to be experienced by any person, whatever their age, who finds themselves acting as a carer. However, while young carers face many of the same problems as other carers, they also face some which are specific to them alone, either on account of their age or because of the lack of status and power which young people have in society. One obvious example (which is identified by a number of the contributions in this collection and which we return to below) is the relationship between young carers and adults who occupy positions of professional responsibility.

Schooling

Unless adequate alternative education is being organised for them, young carers under the school leaving age should be attending school. However, studies of young carers have shown that many of these children and young people miss quite significant periods of their schooling. The 1995 national YCRG study, for example, found that one in four young carers was missing school. Another study found poor school attendance in 43% of children who were caring for sick or disabled parents.

It is understandable why a young carer, looking after a seriously ill member of the family, may decide that their priority is to stay at home rather than go to school. We could imagine how, in this sort of situation, the daily school routines could seem irrelevant to the 'real' issues, perhaps literally of life and death, at home. Even a teacher who is well informed about the home situation of their pupil and is sensitive to the issues facing young carers may not necessarily seem to have very much to offer.

Unfortunately, too, this sort of teacher is likely to be very much the exception. Generally speaking, schools have been slower than social services departments to get to grips with the reality that some children are undertaking caring relationships at home. According to one recent report, one in three young carers believes that their teachers are not aware that they are a carer. In this situation, it is not surprising if young carers are accused of being lazy or indolent when they fail to deliver homework on time, or start yawning in class.

Even where the teachers are aware of the situation and are well-meaning, their actions may be inappropriate. A 1993 study of young carers in Nottinghamshire reported the case of one young carer, 'Miriam', who was missing a great deal of school in order to look after her mother who had MS. The following extract is given in Miriam's own words:

> The teacher asked me who did the cleaning up in the house and I said that I did it and she asked me if I wanted to have some of my classmates to come round and help me clean up. I said no thank you. Then she bought my mother a plant. She got the class to club together and bought my mother a plant!

If teachers are sometimes less understanding than one might wish, the attitudes of young carers' fellow school students may also be problematic. Surveys of young carers have found that many children and young people do not tell their classmates, or even friends, that they are looking after someone. Not surprisingly, this is more likely if they are caring for somebody who has a mental health problem or is misusing alcohol or drugs or, especially, if the person has HIV/AIDS.

There is also some evidence that young carers may be more likely to experience bullying at school. The Princess Royal Trust for Carers, which has a network of more than 80 carers centres around the country, looked at this upsetting subject in its report *Too Much to Take On*. This found that 71% of a group of 240 young carers had been bullied at school (bullying is defined as verbal, physical or emotional abuse). For young carers who were the main carers at home (as opposed to those who shared caring responsibilities), the likelihood of being bullied seems to be greater: 80% of the children and young people in this category who were surveyed said that they experienced some form of bullying, and almost half of this group said that they were bullied most days.

This report does not completely clarify whether young carers are particularly likely to be singled out for bullying, perhaps because other children sense that they are in some way different from their peers. It may be simply that bullying is such an endemic problem in schools that most children may experience it, whether they are young carers or not.

Schools and educational authorities have procedures in place which are intended to prevent non-attendance and truancy by pupils. In the case of young carers, the response of the school authorities, and especially of the education welfare officers who have the front-line task of following up non-attendance, seems to fall into one of two categories.

On the one hand, there are distressing accounts of young carers' parents being taken to court, at a time when they or members of the family were battling with major health crises. The Nottinghamshire study already mentioned reports the example of 'Jimmy', whose father was dying of a brain tumour:

> The education authorities investigated Jimmy's case and took his father to court. Three months later they took Jimmy to court. He told them his father was very ill, but he said that as far as they were concerned his father was getting better. They put Jimmy on probation. He still didn't attend school and eventually he had a home visit: 'I did let them in, they saw my dad say for about five minutes and then they walked out, never to be heard from again.'

Perhaps because they realise that using the courts is hardly the best way of helping young carers receive their education, the second approach of school authorities tends to be one of collusion in young people's absences. Reading young carers' own accounts of their school experiences (including some of those published in this collection) what is striking is how much time many of them have taken off school – and how little the schools seem to have done in response. It is as though the schools are prepared to tolerate grudgingly the necessity for young carers to be at home, but are unable to think beyond this to contemplate other ways of ensuring that children do not miss out on the education which is their right. It may also be that the pressure for good league table results is encouraging schools not to try too hard with pupils who they suspect will not achieve the best grades.

The government's National Strategy for Carers considers the role of schools in relation to young carers and makes a number of proposals. In particular, the Strategy says:

> The Government will draw schools' attention to effective prac-
> tice in meeting the needs of pupils who are young carers, for
> example, through link arrangements with young carers' pro-
> jects... Schools might find it helpful to have one member of staff
> to act as a link between young carers, the education welfare
> service, social services and young carers' projects.

We shall return to this issue again in the following chapter.

Young carers' own health

Researchers who have talked to young carers have drawn attention to the possible implications of caring for children's own health.

Caring can cause physical health problems. The risk in particular of back pain among young carers who have the task of lifting or carrying adults has been highlighted by Sarah Hill, in an article *The physical effects of caring on children*. She describes the case of one young carer, David, as follows:

> David is 12; he lives with his mother, Sue, and his father, John.
> Sue had a stroke four months ago. She cannot walk and tasks
> such as washing, dressing or using the toilet are impossible
> without a substantial amount of physical assistance, including
> lifting... John works shifts and so can be out of the house at all
> hours leaving David to help his mother alone. The family has
> been given a hoist but no one has tried to show David how to use
> it. He has tried to use the hoist but, worried that his mother may
> fall, he prefers to lift her by himself. David has not been taught
> how to lift. David is now regularly taking time off school for
> 'back problems'.

One problem seems to be that social workers and community nurses do not feel that it is appropriate to show children and young people the right way to lift people, on the legitimate grounds that they feel that young people should not be doing this work. This is understandable, but does not help at all unless young carers are provided with an adequate alternative.

It may also be that some professionals fail to understand the work which young carers are performing. Sarah Hill mentions the case of the social worker 'who could not bring himself to believe that a ten year old boy was carrying his father up the stairs until he actually saw it happen'. She concludes her article: 'It seems highly likely that a number of young carers will go on to experience back pain as adults. Some may even become disabled. It is ironic that the same organisation and structures that are failing young carers today will be those that have responsibility for caring for them in the future as disabled adults.'

However, young carers may be even more at risk of stress and of mental health problems. As Chris Dearden and Saul Becker point out in *Young Carers in the UK*, caring can be very emotionally worrying and stressful: 'For children, this stress may be caused by worries not simply about their relative's long-term future, e.g. the deterioration of parental health, the possible death of a close relative or hospitalisation, but also their own future if anything should happen to their parent.'

Future careers and adult life

So what happens when children and young people who have spent their youth in a caring relationship grow up and become adults? Do they look back and, in the words of one Australian report, feel 'all cared out'?

As a consequence of the development in public awareness of the issue of young carers in recent years, some adults who were themselves young carers have taken the opportunity to look back on their childhood and assess its effects on their lives. For example Lyn Shore, who now works with adult carers, has written in the *Journal of Young Carers Work* about her own time as a young carer, looking after a disabled mother:

It is thirty years since my young caring ended but it still affects my lifecourse. My subsequent relationships and life choices have been profoundly influenced by it. There have been positive and negative outcomes, but I suspect there might have been more positives and fewer negatives had intervention been available which helped our family understand and manage our situation better. It is encouraging that today's young carers are visible…

A recent report published by the Children's Society tried to explore just what might be the 'concealed consequences' for adult life chances of being a young carer. The 1999 report, *On Small Shoulders* (by J. Frank, C. Tatum and S. Tucker), is based on a survey of about 60 former young carers, and the conclusions are stark: according to the authors, caring as a young person 'can have profound social, psychological and emotional effects in later life'.

About 70% of those surveyed had long-term psychological effects from their time as a young carer, with those who had cared for a family member with mental health or alcohol abuse being most vulnerable. About half had had some form of counselling, and about 40% felt their own mental health had been directly affected. A smaller number commented that their physical health in adulthood had suffered. About three-quarters of the group surveyed also felt, looking back, that their education had been affected.

Many of the former young carers thought that their experiences in childhood had directly influenced their career choices and encouraged them to make their work in one of a number of caring professions. This phenomenon, which is also apparent from the recent report by Chris Dearden and Saul Becker already mentioned, *Growing Up Caring*, can be assessed in two ways. On the one hand, it may mean that former young carers find that they can turn the skills they have acquired into paid work. On the other, it could mean that their career choices have been unhealthily limited, for example by an absence of educational qualifications. The authors of *Growing Up Caring* summarise this point as follows, but also make an interesting additional observation:

> There may be a danger of young carers moving into 'caring' jobs or professions because they feel these are the only skills they have to offer. Many of these jobs will be low paid with few prospects. However, while they may be lacking formal qualifications, the young people had many other qualities which employers would value, such as organisational skills, independence, maturity, etc. Currently these qualities are not validated or accredited in any way which employers would recognise.

In fact, the experience of having been a young carer can give the adult insights which should be valued by the whole of society. One person who has spoken movingly of her childhood, growing up with a father who had schizophrenia, is Dr Lynne Jones, who is now a Birmingham MP. His illness meant, among other things, that she spent the evening before one of her A level exams waiting for several hours on her grandmother's doorstep for her grandmother to return home; because of her father's state of mind, her mother had not wanted to return to their own house that evening. Her experiences mirror those of today's young carers, including the social stigma of parental ill health (particularly mental illness), the lack of help and support and the lack of consultation with children about their own needs.

Lynne Jones attributes her own success in later life to the key role played by her mother. She adds that she now is prepared to talk publicly about her childhood as a way of raising awareness about mental health issues and schizophrenia.

Poverty and social exclusion

Family poverty seems to be an almost inevitable corollary of family ill health and disability. Even previously affluent households become poor if their income suddenly drops, or if they have to rely on state benefits for any considerable period. A focus on the practical caring work carried out by young carers should not mean that we overlook this aspect of their lives. The report *Growing Up Caring* puts the point forcibly:

> Almost all of the young people lived in families that were in receipt of welfare benefits. Many were living in poverty... Half of the respondents lived with lone parents. The combination of lone parenthood and illness or disability makes entire families vulnerable to poverty and social exclusion.

Society is based on the principle that children and young people are financially dependent on their parents, which of course remains the case even where those children are caring for ill or disabled parents. This means that children share with other members of the household any financial privations which come as a consequence of ill health and disability.

There are no welfare benefit payments which take into account the work which young carers are undertaking, for while Invalid Care Allowance is payable to adult carers giving regular and substantial care, it is not payable to young people until they reach 16, and then not if they remain in full-time education or enter employment. Younger carers' contribution to the care of ill or disabled members of their family (and thus to 'care in the community' for these people) remains unrecognised in any formal sense by the benefits system. This is not to argue that the answer would be for younger carers to receive their own benefit entitlement; as we make clear in the next chapter, the preferred approach to this, as to other issues raised by the presence of young people undertaking caring responsibilities, is to tackle it at the family level – or, of course, to prevent it occurring in the first place. However, the feeling of financial disempowerment which is common to many young people may be reinforced in the case of young carers, especially those who are taking on money-management responsibilities as part of their caring work.

Beyond age 16, the situation remains problematic. Recent years have seen welfare benefit entitlements for this age group increasingly withdrawn, as young people are encouraged to remain in education or training and under the responsibility of their parents.

While this public policy strategy may or may not be appropriate in general for young people, it can hit particularly harshly those young people who are in caring relationships. *Growing Up Caring* offered the following comment on this issue: 'The benefit system does not recognise the particular needs of ill or disabled parents who have adolescent children. Assumptions are made regarding family/parental responsibilities to support their children for longer and longer periods of time...'

A similar observation can be made about the removal of further and higher education grants and allowances. Students who feel unable to complete courses because of family illnesses are particularly penalised.

Information and support

Discussion of welfare benefits leads appropriately to a final point, that there is an urgent need to ensure that young carers have access to the information they need.

Welfare benefits are a notoriously complex area, where appropriate information can be difficult to find, for adults as much as for young people. However there are also other areas of young carers' lives where 'adult' information which young carers need is not adequately shared with them or given in appropriate ways. This is particularly true of medical information. Unfortunately, the comments of two young carers quoted in a national newspaper suggest that medical professionals are not good at remembering to talk to young people. One described a visit from a nurse in this way:

'[She] came once and that was it... She didn't even talk to me.'

Another said:

'You are ignored – it's like you're not there... Nobody wants to know what I want.'

Interviews with young carers suggest that in many cases they have only a hazy knowledge of the medical diagnosis of the person they are caring for and are not being given the information they need and have a right to expect.

The case of Jimmy was mentioned above, when we looked at his relationship with school authorities. He also had an unfortunate relationship with those who could have given him the medical information he needed to cope with his father's terminal illness. The study *Children who Care* by Jo Aldridge and Saul Becker reported this as follows:

> He wanted to care for his father and did so against many odds (socio-economic deprivation, lack of support, prosecution), but no one had provided him with a medical prognosis in relation to his father's condition. Although the doctors and specialists may not have been able to predict exactly what the effects of his father's brain tumour might have been, they could have indicated the *possible* effects – medical staff could have engaged Jimmy in discussions about the possible outcomes of his father's condition. However, as Jimmy said: 'The fits, I wasn't told anything of the sort. That was the worst thing. No one said fits.' (Jimmy's father's first fit occurred when he was driving the family car – Jimmy was in the passenger seat at the time).

There is an onus on primary health care professionals, particularly GPs and district nurses (but also specialist workers such as community psychiatric nurses), to ensure that young carers are not left at this sort of level of ignorance. Admittedly, the issue of patient confidentiality has to be taken into account. Just as teenagers visiting a GP should be able to do so if they wish without their parents' knowledge, so parents with an illness or disability may not want others in their family, including their children, to be aware of their medical condition.

Nevertheless, the issue of confidentiality should not be used as a convenient shield for medical professionals to retreat behind. It is, after all, quite easy for the GP or community nurse to explain to their patient why it would be advisable to give the young carer appropriate medical information, and indeed to offer to do so themselves. Knowledge, even of unpleasant things, can be reassuring, and it is patronising to imagine that children and young people are too young to know what is going on in their families.

The problem, in practice, seems to be that GPs in particular are used to seeing and treating just the individual who is disabled or suffering ill health. This process does not lend itself to taking into account the full family context. A simple question asked by the GP of their patient in this situation – Who is helping to care for you? – might be a trigger to identify the needs of young carers and to enable action to be taken on their behalf.

A similar criticism can be levelled at social care professionals who fail to involve young carers, particularly in discussions and formal assessments of the needs of the person being cared for. Though the issue of young carers has been on the agenda for social care professionals for several years (and young carers received their own entitlement to a needs assessment in the 1995 Carers Act), social workers and others may still need to be reminded of the need to work sensitively and in partnership with a young carer. The tradition in social services departments of handling adult casework separately from child casework may be an obstacle here.

The inequality in power which inevitably exists between the adult professional and the young carer also needs to be recognised and overcome. Social workers have powers granted from the state to take children into care. A number of studies of young carers have shown that some young carers and their families are fearful of receiving the attentions of social workers, because they fear that this will indeed be the outcome.

Ensuring that young carers have the information they need is an essential step towards empowering them, so that they are not forced to play the role of 'little victim'. But we can extend this point: the requirement is to provide support for both young carers and their families, so that there are neither 'young victims', nor, indeed, 'older victims' in the household.

Chapter 2

Young Carers
and Public Policy

The General Assembly of the United Nations adopted its Convention on
the Rights of the Child on 20 November 1989. The wording of the Convention which was agreed on that occasion had taken ten years to draft,
and the working group charged with the task was itself building on earlier work which the League of Nations had begun when a declaration on
children's rights was adopted back in 1924.

The UN Convention on the Rights of the Child does not occupy a
very prominent place in the popular consciousness in Britain. Nevertheless the Convention is the nearest thing there is to a commonly
agreed statement by the world community on its obligations to its children and young people. It runs to a total of 54 articles. Several of these
are directly relevant to the position of young carers. Article 31, for
example, recognises the right of children 'to rest and leisure' and
to engage in play and recreational activities appropriate to their age.
Articles 28 and 29 lay down the right of the child to education towards
'the development of the child's personality, talents and mental and
physical abilities to their fullest potential'. Article 24 is about the child's
right to the highest attainable standard of health. Article 16 sets out a
child's right to privacy. Article 12 stresses the right of children to have
their own views taken into account. Other Articles cover such areas as
family life, responsibilities of parents, children's right to information
and much else. This chapter, however, will be concerned with the implications of Article 4.

Article 4 describes the responsibility which rests on each state
under the Convention. States are instructed to 'undertake all appropriate legislative, administrative, and other measures' to ensure that the
children's rights identified in the Convention are protected. States are
told that, when it comes to children's economic, social and cultural
rights, they should 'undertake such measures to the maximum extent of
their available resources'.

So how does the government in Britain, which ratified the Convention on the Rights of the Child in 1991, measure up when it comes to protecting the rights of the country's young carers? What changes to public policy might be needed to improve the present situation?

Young carers in the UK: the government response

The government's publication in 1999 of its National Strategy for Carers marked something of a landmark in official recognition of the important role played in society by those who care for others. For young carers, the National Strategy was particularly significant, since the needs of these children and young people was considered important enough to merit separate consideration. One chapter of the National Strategy looks specifically at the issues facing young carers.

The National Strategy identifies nine frequent effects on children and young people of providing care. These are:

- Problems at school, with completing homework and in getting qualifications
- Isolation from other children of the same age and from other family members
- Lack of time for play, sport or leisure activities
- Conflict between the needs of the person they are helping and their own needs, leading to feelings of guilt and resentment
- Feeling that there is nobody there for them, that professionals do not listen to them and are working only with the adult
- Lack of recognition, praise, or respect for their contribution
- Feeling that they are different from other children and unable to be part of a group
- Feeling that no one else understands their experience
- Problems moving into adulthood, especially with finding work, their own home, and establishing relationships

The government goes on in its National Strategy to pledge improved support for young carers, and offers a number of concrete proposals with implications for local authority social services departments, the education service and the health service. We will look in more detail at these in a moment. To understand the context of the National Strategy for Carers' chapter on young carers, however, it is necessary first to go back ten or more years.

The start of the 1990s saw a major reform in the way in which the state intervened in the lives of disabled, infirm and chronically ill people. The guidelines for what became known as 'care in the community' were laid in the influential Griffiths report of 1988, which was followed by legislation two years later, in the NHS and Community Care Act. The community care reforms actually came fully into effect by 1993.*

These changes put family carers at the centre of the 'care in the community' approach. This strategy involved an attempt to move away from the institutionalising of ill and disabled people, which could be welcomed by, among others, disabled people themselves, especially those who had increasingly been articulating an agenda based on a disability rights perspective. But conveniently the new approach also satisfied the New Right thinking of the Thatcher and Major administrations, to the extent that it represented a reduction in state provision of services and an opportunity to save on government expenditure on social care and welfare.

Under the new regime, local authority social services departments maintain a regulatory and financing responsibility, but are less involved in service delivery, which may be undertaken by private and voluntary sector organisations. The key event in this process is the assessment of needs of the person for whom community care is required, which social services departments undertake. Following this, in theory at least, an individual care plan is drawn up, setting out how those needs will be met. The major aim is to enable people to continue living in their own homes within the community.

Where does this leave the carer, on whom much of the unpaid caring work is likely to fall? In theory, under the NHS and Community Care legislation, carers were supposed to be consulted and involved in the process of needs assessment and care plan development. In practice, many carers have argued that, certainly in the first few years of the implementation of community care, this involvement did not take place. Too many social services departments remained locked in a traditional service-led culture.

More substantively, carers and their organisations criticised the NHS and Community Care legislation for failing adequately to meet their own needs. But if this was true for adult carers, for young carers

---

*Legislation referred to in this chapter applies specifically to England and Wales; the position of young carers under Scottish law is different. Scotland has parallel legislation to England and Wales.

the position was even less satisfactory. Their interests and needs were not covered or protected at all under the legislation, which was intended specifically for adults.

This omission is perhaps understandable, since at the stage when the Act was passed there was little general recognition of the existence and role of young carers in society. As awareness of young carers grew in the 1990s, some social care professionals looked instead to another important piece of legislation, the Children Act 1989, to see if this could be used to offer support for children and young people who were taking on caring responsibilities.

The Children Act framework gave local authorities a duty to 'safeguard and promote the welfare of children within their areas who are in need'. Could young carers be categorised in this way? A small number of authorities (11 out of 71 surveyed, according to a Department of Health study in 1996) did adopt this approach, which had the advantage of enabling social services departments to offer a range of services to the young carers and their families. But while in theory this approach offered professional recognition to young carers for the work they were undertaking at home, in practice the 'children in need' tag was problematic. Families may – sometimes justifiably – fear that social services intervention can lead to the children being taken into care.

A better way forward seemed to arrive with the passing of the Carers (Recognition and Services) Act 1995. Since this Act applied to all carers regardless of age, for the first time effective official recognition was given to young carers. For the first time young carers' own needs could be formally taken into account.

In essence, the Carers Act entitles carers providing (or about to provide) a substantial amount of caring on a regular basis to have their own needs assessed at the time when the person they are caring for is having their own formal needs assessment. The result of the carer's needs assessment has to be taken into account when social services draw up the care plan of services to be made available.

Young carers' specific needs were also considered in the Department of Health Practice Guide which accompanied the Act and which was circulated to social services departments. These guidelines pointed out that the denial of proper educational and social opportunities to young carers could have harmful consequences, and went on to state that 'the provision of community care services should ensure that young carers are not expected to carry inappropriate levels of caring responsibilities'.

Implementing the legislation

Legislation is important, both because it gives public bodies access to financial resources and because it provides an overall official framework for approaching an issue. But there is of course a world of difference between the passing by Parliament of an Act and its implementation at the grassroots. We therefore need to consider what the effect of this legislation has actually been for young carers.

One problem is that the Carers Act has a major limitation: the assessment of a carer's needs takes place only if carers themselves request that it happens. This means that carers have to know their rights and entitlements under the Act, and understand that it is potentially in their interests to take up this particular entitlement.

Surveys of *adult* carers have identified the low take-up of needs assessments. A 1997 survey of 1,600 carers undertaken by the Carers National Association, for example, revealed that only 18% had requested an assessment.

It is not surprising, therefore, if the evidence points to very few young carers having had formal needs assessments. The 1997 survey undertaken by members of the Young Carers Research Group (YCRG) already mentioned (published in 1998 in *Young Carers in the UK*) found that only 249 of the 2,303 young carers surveyed were in this position. As the authors pointed out, this figure was low considering that the survey was of young carers already known to young carers projects:

> Given the relatively low age of the young carers in contact with projects (the average age is just 12), and that many are involved in intimate and other caring tasks or responsibilities (indicative of substantial or regular care), and that many children seem to be experiencing negative effects on their own development or transition to adulthood, then we might have expected a far greater incidence of assessments than is the case.

There is another potential weakness in the way that the Carers Act 1995 is working. While the Act imposes on local authorities the procedure for undertaking if requested a needs assessment of a young carer, it does *not* oblige the authority actually to provide any of the services which the needs assessment may show to be necessary. In other words, if the budget is not there to supply these services, young carers' needs may continue to be neglected.

In practice, in the minority of cases where needs assessments of young carers have taken place, the evidence seems to show that the outcome is usually positive. As *Young Carers in the UK* shows, services were either introduced or increased after an assessment, and most children and their families were satisfied with the outcome.

The issue of needs assessment remains vital, therefore, when considering public policy towards young carers. The 1999 National Strategy for Carers made the following comment:

> Under the Carers (Recognition and Services) Act 1995, young carers can ask for an assessment of their needs. But many are not aware that this is possible. Some local authorities are reluctant to advertise this fact because of their concern about raising expectations. With the help of the voluntary sector, the statutory services should ensure that young carers are not expected to carry inappropriate levels of caring responsibility. To achieve this, disabled or ill parents need support to maintain their independence and to carry out their parenting responsibilities...

The encounter between the young carer, their family and the social services professional can still be an uneasy one but at least the development of a legislative framework for community care in recent years should mean that a social worker or social care professional has some understanding of the nature of the young carer's experience.

In 2000 the government, through the Department of Health, introduced a new framework for assessing all children who become known to social services for whatever reason. This framework requires those assessing children, especially children in need, to consider three 'domains' – the child's developmental needs, the ability of the parent(s) to provide adequate parenting, and family and environmental factors. Future assessments of young carers should take into account their needs, their development, the needs and capacities of their ill or disabled parents, and environmental factors such as poverty or poor housing. This should, in due course, result in better assessments of existing young carers, the prevention of some children taking on heavy caring responsibilities, and support for the wider family. It is an excellent step in the right direction.

Such improvements are less in evidence, however, in the case of other professionals who deal with young carers, such as teachers or health care workers. In particular, there may be a lack of close cross-agency links.

The National Strategy for Carers looked particularly at the situation regarding schools. Chapter 1 considered in some detail issues surrounding young carers' education and schooling, and noted in passing the suggestion in the National Strategy that schools should provide a young carers' 'link person', responsible for liaising with the education welfare service, social services and young carers projects. According to the National Strategy, 'the person could benefit from getting to know others who can help young carers and what services are available in the area to meet their needs'.

The government has also attempted to brief head teachers and education welfare officers on the particular needs of young carers, in a guidance note circulated for consultation early in 1999. There is official recognition, however, that more could be done. The National Strategy pledges to 'promote awareness of young carers in schools through ensuring that teaching on Personal, Social and Health Education includes references to young carers', and it also promises to improve awareness about young carers during teachers' initial training and subsequently after qualification.

This is all commendable, though cynics may argue that schools are currently struggling under a heavy workload imposed by central government which is likely to mean that most head teachers and governors have their minds on other matters. Furthermore, most academic research and writing on young carers has emerged from social policy departments rather than from education departments, so that there has not been the same level of debate in educational circles.

To a large extent, many of the same comments apply also to the health service. GPs, community nurses and other primary health care workers need to be better briefed on the issues raised by young carers. Here the National Strategy for Carers is disappointingly brief, simply pledging – as it did in the case of teachers – to 'improve awareness training'.

The young carers projects

The message from the National Strategy for Carers is that more can, and should, be done for young carers. One very concrete achievement has, however, already come from the work of the pioneer researchers and campaigners on the issue. This is the creation of a network of more than 100 young carers projects and groups.

The development of young carers projects has been striking. Less than ten years ago, only two such groups were operating. By 1998, when a detailed handbook of projects was published, 110 could be listed, with a geographical spread from Kirkcaldy to Truro, Ballymena to Thetford.

These young carers projects inevitably differ from town to town, but share many characteristics. They are normally funded from statutory sources but run by the voluntary sector. Major national charities such as Barnardo's, NCH Action for Children, the Children's Society, Crossroads and the Princess Royal Trust for Carers are among the organisations involved. The projects also tend to be generic in their approach, offering help and support for all young carers in their area of operation. However, a project specifically for black young carers has operated in Manchester and another for Asian children and young people has been run in London, while in Leeds a young carers project was set up specifically for children caring for people with mental health problems.

What do the young carers projects hope to achieve? Saul Becker, Jo Aldridge and Chris Dearden in their 1998 book *Young Carers and their Families* put it like this:

> Although working with families is an important aspect of the work of these projects, their primary focus is on supporting children as carers. In this respect most projects offer counselling, advocacy and befriending services specifically for young carers. Some of this counselling and befriending work is provided on an informal basis (someone to talk to, a confidante) although some projects provide or arrange more formal services where applicable. Advocacy is considered an essential service by many projects since many young carers – indeed many children – are unaware of their rights. Project workers can therefore work with them or act on their behalf to try and secure their rights under existing legislation...
>
> Around 80% of projects arrange leisure activities for young carers. Indeed, in many cases these are the services that young carers value most...

For children and young people facing major responsibilities at home, the opportunity to come together for indoor activities, or go out for a group trip, is highly prized – a 'thumbs up night', in the words of one young carer, who was reporting on a Christmas meal out at Pizzaland.

The authors of *Young Carers and their Families* conclude with this assessment:

> Mixing with other young carers can serve to validate the young caring experience and reassure children that they are not alone. Although project workers stress the fact that young carers rarely

sit around discussing their experiences or home life, during interviews many young carers have said that it can be comforting to know that, among other young carers, there is no need to explain their circumstances and their feelings will be understood.

The National Strategy for Carers makes a very similar point in its own positive assessment of the role of young carers projects: 'These projects can provide relief from the isolation faced by children who are carers. They are places where the young can go for advice, information and support or leisure activities and can share experiences with other young carers.'

Notwithstanding the growth of the past few years, there are some major towns and cities in Britain which do not yet provide young carers projects. Any strategy for improving the experience of children and young people undertaking caring responsibilities would need to address – or so it would seem – the current gaps in the network. However, despite the vitally important work which many young carers projects clearly do, a question mark hangs over the future of the concept.

There are two reasons for this. Firstly, there is the issue of funding. Many young carers initiatives have been financed on a project basis, typically for a set period of years, rather than having their costs met from core funding budgets. Project funding is a familiar, and often convenient, way of piloting new ideas and initiatives, but it does raise the problem of what happens when the initial project funding runs out. As early as 1997, this was already beginning to worry several young carers groups.

The funding for young carers projects has in practice come from a variety of sources. The situation in 1997 was reviewed by the authors of *Young Carers and their Families*:

Approximately 40% of projects received part of their core funding from joint finance (a mixture of social services and health authority funding), more than 40% from social services alone and slightly less than one-fifth from health authorities. Approximately one-fifth received some core funding from charities or voluntary organisations while only four projects received part of their core funding from education. In Britain the introduction of the National Lottery has provided an additional potential source of funding, with nine projects receiving core funding. Corporate funding has been low...

The same report went on to comment that fewer than half of the 106 established projects in 1997 considered future funding to be 'likely' or 'very likely' and that 52 were unsure about their financial futures. In fact, although a number of groups have disappeared, it is clear three years on that there has been no major collapse in the funding of young carers projects – at least not yet. Nevertheless, the constant worry about future funding drains staff morale, and also means that resources which should be directed at the key work of engaging with young carers gets diverted into fundraising tasks.

If finance is one concern, the future of the young carers project network faces another challenge, this time from a much less obvious direction. Some people, including those who would argue passionately that society needs to give more resources to help people who are chronically ill or have disabilities, feel that the emphasis on young carers groups has been a mistake. We should be looking in another direction entirely.

Children's rights, disability rights

To understand the background to what, at times, has been a heated dispute, it is necessary to return to something discussed in the previous chapter.

The critique of the traditional view of disability which has been developed over the past 20 or 30 years by disabled people and their supporters has had both social and political consequences of some importance. It has involved a sharp attack on what could be conveniently described as the 'does he take sugar?' approach to disability. Such an approach, the disability rights movement has pointed out, not only demeans but also disempowers those people in our society who have disabilities.

The power and vitality of the disability movement was there for all to see in the street protests which followed the initial unsuccessful attempts to introduce a disability bill in Parliament. London police, it was clear, were inexperienced in the appropriate way of removing wheelchair-using demonstrators from under the front wheels of London buses. But while the eventual successful passing into law of the Disability Discrimination Act in 1995 could be seen to mark a watershed for disability rights in Britain, disability campaigners would argue that the battles are by no means over. Some of the tensions of recent years in long-established and powerful establishment charities such as the Royal National Institute for the Blind and the Royal National Institute for Deaf People focus exactly on this issue – are charities like these there to be run *for* disabled people, or *by* them? Empowerment, or continued patronage?

Given this background, it is not surprising if some disability rights activists looked at what was happening with young carers, and decided that they were not very happy with what they saw. Richard Olsen of the University of Leicester has described it like this:

> If the trend in policy and practice was perceived as one emphasising 'caring for the carers' rather than addressing the barriers that disabled people face, then this sudden interest in labelling the children of some disabled parents 'young carers' was bound to engender hostility... If some disabled people were angry at seeing resources directed at supporting carers rather than, as they saw it, at promoting independence and control on the part of disabled people themselves, then the suggestion that their children should be supported as their carers in this way was always likely to be inflammatory...

As Richard Olsen goes on to point out, the young carer approach 'involved giving the kind of rights to children (to consultation about a parental condition, to information about parental treatment, to a separate assessment of need, to property such as washing machines, and so on) that most non-disabled parents would find at the very least undermining of their parental role if granted to their own children'.

In other words, perhaps with the best of motives the emphasis on young carers' rights was once again leading to the familiar situation where the disabled person found themselves disempowered, belittled and discriminated against.

Opposition to the notion that the rights of young carers should take precedence over the rights of disabled people developed during the later 1990s and was not confined to the academic sphere. Rick Howell, who had been project manager of the young carers project in Macclesfield for three years until the funding ran out in 1998, contributed a thoughtful piece to the *Journal of Young Carers Work* reflecting on his experiences. He described how one of his social care colleagues had challenged the work which his project, and other young carers projects, had been trying to do:

> He said that young carers projects had created a myth, that to respond to young carers you needed to have a project and be experts... Young carers projects were perpetuating the idea that

children who were carers are a new welfare category and some-
how different from other young people. He contended that this
was dangerous, because at best it undermined the idea of main-
streaming responses and at worst further alienates and stigma-
tises parents affected by ill health and disabilities. He suggested
that at the centre of many *families'* difficulties were issues such
as low income, transport problems and inflexible support.

Rick Howell went on to make his own assessment of the role of his, and
other, young carers projects:

> The issue of young carers is 'moving on' and while projects still
> have a role in the future there is a need to look at new direc-
> tions... Do projects make a difference? I would say yes, a big yes
> they do make a difference to the lives of many families *and*
> provide an essential focus when trying to build recognition
> and services. *But*, are they sustainable or acceptable as service
> providers in their current form? Are they the best way to
> make a long-term difference? These questions are less easy to
> answer...

Underlying the dispute between the disability rights and young carer
perspectives it was possible to see two theoretical approaches and belief
systems chafing against each other. The background to the disability
rights perspective has been set out above. On the other side was an
approach which came from an emphasis on children's rights, and which
could offer its own powerful critique, of the disempowerment of
children in an adult-dominated and controlled world.

But the dispute was never quite so clear-cut as this might imply.
Looked at from the outside, the two positions appear to have a lot in
common with each other and would seem to be natural allies, particularly against other, more conservative, philosophies and practices. And,
in reality, the arguments advanced by many of those researching and
working with young carers, even in the early years of the 1990s, were
considerably more subtle than an exclusive belief in the rights of young
carers.

Towards a family-centred approach

By 1998, members of the YCRG (in their book *Young Carers and their
Families*) were announcing the arrival of what they hoped would be a
new way forward, a new paradigm which would replace the old

medicalised view of disability and which could transcend the disability
rights and young carer approaches:

> A fourth paradigm, a family perspective, has emerged as a direct
> consequence of the debate between the rights of disabled people
> and the rights of children who care, and is congruent with the
> principle of the government's refocusing strategy which empha-
> sises prevention in a family context as opposed to protection.

This 'whole family' approach argues that offering support either to the
young carer or the family member who is ill or disabled is not sufficient:
support for the whole family is essential.

The recent YCRG report *Growing Up Caring* elaborates the arguments further:

> Young carers' independence cannot be separated from their
> parent's independence. It is not possible to have true independ-
> ence for one without independence for the other. Ill and dis-
> abled parents need to be supported as parents as well as disabled
> people, so that they can achieve personal independence and
> control over their own lives and provide the kind and quality of
> parenting to their children that they wish for. This will enable
> many families to prevent children from having to take on caring
> responsibilities in the first place, especially in the absence of any
> alternatives.

Two interesting points emerge from this extract. First, there is an
emphasis, which was not present in earlier writings, on helping
disabled or ill parents fulfil their role *as parents*. This was one of the
issues which Richard Olsen raised in the extract quoted above. The
argument is that disabled or ill parents should have the right to state
support not only to enable them to meet their own needs but also to
meet their parental responsibilities towards their children – otherwise
they are implicitly being patronised and demeaned.

To summarise the argument, the 'whole family' approach looks to
replace the one-sided caring which many young carers currently undertake with a more natural, two-way process, where parents (whether
disabled or ill, or not) are also enabled to care for their children. In other
words, the desired aim is to reach towards the sort of natural exchange
of help and affection which reinforces family relationships and which
should be a mark of a successfully functioning family.

The second, related, argument raised in the passage above is that – if this parenting support is provided – it will help to prevent children and young people from being forced into a caring relationship in the first place.

The question of the extent to which young carers should be caring at all underlies much research and writing on young carers, and it is clearly a difficult one. On the one hand, young carers have made it clear when interviewed that they would not necessarily welcome professional intervention if the result was a break-up of the family or the enforced hospitalisation of the person they are caring for. Any move to remove existing caring responsibilities from young people could itself be construed as patronising, forcing them back into a childhood role which they have left behind.

On the other hand, nobody would argue that children or young people should undertake some of the things which are revealed in interviews with young carers and the literature written about them – including some of the extracts in this book. Whatever the issues at the 'softer' end of caring, there is a clear and straightforward consensus when it comes to the 'harder' end – particularly the sort of intimate personal care which some young carers undertake for their parents.

The 'whole family' approach was already being recommended by the government in 1996. A letter from the Department of Health to directors of social services departments states: 'Where the disabled person is a parent, it is essential that the community care assessment focuses on the family and considers how to support the parent and recognise the needs of any young carers.' The letter was accompanied by an action checklist, with nine points:

- Start with the needs of the family/disabled or ill parent, and see what needs remain for the child.
- Work with the child as part of the family unit.
- Acknowledge the rights of the child including the right to information, to be listened to and to stop physically caring.
- Recognise that poverty and disabling environments, services and attitudes can limit adults' ability to parent.
- Acknowledge the distinction between *parenting* and *parental activity*.
- Recognise that time spent in counselling, talking and therapeutic work can prevent inappropriate and expensive crisis responses.
- Focus more on support for children in need rather than on protection of children at risk.

- Acknowledge young carers' legitimate concerns about profession-als' attitudes and insensitivity and their fear of professional inter-vention.
- Remember 'families do their best'. Start with the family's solution and work with any dilemmas and contradictions.

This remarkably enlightened checklist, if properly adopted and funded, would do much to remove many of the problems and concerns which have emerged in relation to young carers and their caring responsibili-ties

If a family-centred approach is to be adopted, however, it will mean re-examining a number of aspects of current work with young carers. Indeed the YCRG report *Growing Up Caring* issues a clarion call for 'a fundamental change to the existing structures for young carers services'.

Some young carers projects are already beginning to ponder the way forward and are redefining themselves as projects for families. Mavis Crawforth, for example, is project manager for Choices for Families in Hull, which grew out of work in the city undertaken with young carers. Writing in the *Journal of Young Carers Work* in 1999, she described the work of the new project:

> Disabled parents whose children used the project felt disillu-sioned and isolated and were surprised to hear from their chil-dren that they were meeting other young people living in similar circumstances. At the request of the parents a meeting was facilitated by the project to enable parents to meet others. Those parents who were able to attend quickly established a lot of common ground. By the end of what had been planned as a social event the embryo of a new movement had emerged…
>
> At that first meeting parents had shared with each other how most of what little energies they had was spent on fighting the system in order to (a) gain a better quality of life for them-selves and (b) to have their status as a parent recognised and respected. They were all able to share anecdotal evidence of how they felt their parenting role was or had been undermined…

To sum up, as the YCRG authors of *Growing Up Caring* state:

> Policies and services which identify and respond to the needs of all family members, but in particular those which support ill

or disabled parents to enable them to prevent inappropriate caring roles from developing, will offer the best way forward. This challenges us all to think critically about how services to ill and disabled parents, and to existing young carers, should be structured, what they should do, and how they should fit together

In conclusion

What have we learned about the lives and experiences of young carers, and what responses are appropriate?

Firstly, there are in our midst children and young people – perhaps about 50,000, perhaps more – making sometimes substantial efforts to care for members of their families. The work which adult carers do can too often be forgotten or ignored. The work which *young* carers do is even more likely to be hidden from sight. It is an achievement of all those who have worked over the past ten years and more to highlight the issue that the existence of young carers, and the needs they have, are now much more widely recognised in society.

Young carers perform a spectrum of caring work, including domestic work, emotional support and personal care work. Many young carers really are young – primary school children are involved as often as teenagers. Around one in five is undertaking intimate personal care.

Young carers are receiving a poor deal from schools. Many are missing a worryingly large amount of school, and often education service responses are either inadequately heavy-handed or inadequately lax. Teachers need much greater understanding of the young carer experience. Bullying by other children can also be a problem.

Health professionals too need to be better informed. GPs in particular may be treating the individual ill or disabled patient without pausing to consider the family situation they are in. Young carers' own health can be affected by their caring role.

Young carers and their families are, almost by definition, burdened also by poverty. Inevitably social services budgets are under pressure, so that assessed needs cannot always be met. But too many young carers are in any case not receiving their own needs assessment, which is their entitlement under the Carers Act. In addition, the state benefits system does not recognise the particular needs of ill or disabled parents with teenage children.

Young carers have a right to be given the information they need. They suffer from a double disadvantage when relating to professionals:

as children dealing with adults, and as lay individuals dealing with those who have authority and power.

Young carers develop skills and competencies from their caring work which are not appreciated or recognised. As a consequence many young carers have unnecessarily limited career choices in later life.

The network of young carers groups have performed sterling work at local level, in supporting individual young carers and enabling them to come together collectively. There are, however, still large areas with no young carers groups or projects. Funding is a problem for many existing groups. But young carers groups also need to develop their practice, to take on board the move to a 'whole family' approach.

More generally, social care professionals and others should consider the needs of young carers at the same time as they consider the needs of their parents. Parents have the right to receive support to help them fulfil their role *as parents*. The aim should be to have support in place so that children and young people need no longer cope with the kinds of situation which they describe in the second part of this book. Equally importantly, they deserve to be heard, recognised and respected.

Young Carers in
Their Own Words

Written contributions and interview transcripts –
the latter are indicated by a grey border.

Lucylee, 13

My mum suffers from manic depression and she has a curved spine. She often needs a walking stick and sometimes can't even get out of bed. My parents are divorced. They split up when I was five just before my mum became ill. She said that's what started it off but I don't really know.

My mum re-married about two years later to a man named David. He is very loving and caring and I have accepted him as my new dad. Myself and my brother Tim both look after my mum while my dad is at work. He is a police officer and works long shifts which can be hard for us when mum is really ill.

My mum has to take lots of tablets. Sometimes they don't work and mum becomes very ill. One time she had to change pills and became so sick she fainted. I had to call the doctor and my dad who was at work. When the doctor came he checked my mum and went to get an injection. While he was gone I cried because I was scared but when I heard him come back I stopped. I didn't want him to see me upset so I tried to keep a brave face.

My mum has good days and bad days, it seems most of them are bad but it's nice to see her smile now and again. Tim and I do a lot of the housework and I sometimes have to cook as well as do my home-work. It can get difficult but it's good afterwards knowing I've helped my mum. I enjoy helping my mum, I only wish it could be a bit easier.

Michelle, 10

My mum has epilepsy and MS. My mum is aged 38.

My mum has to take 84 tablets a week. She has to take five in the morning, five at teatime, two at night. Every day of the week. My mum's tablets are called: Lamictal, Carbamazepine, Diazepam.

My mum found out she has MS when she was 25 years old and she found out she had epilepsy when she was 31 years old.

Epilepsy means men/women/boys/girls could start to; stare, shake, and start to bite their clothes, punch, and kick, and sometimes their eyes will roll to the back of the head.

Sometimes little children might cry just like I did when I first saw my mum in an epileptic fit, but now I am used to it. My older brother knows what to do and so does my younger brother, they help me a lot.

My brothers have jobs to do: my younger brother has to get the pillows and get my Nan or uncle. And my older brother has to get everyone out of the house when my mum is in a fit and make a sweet cup of tea.

My younger brother always cries when he sees my mum in a fit. Because he is young my older brother just laughs, he thinks it's funny.

One day my mum had a fit in my school playground and in my school. She had to go to hospital. Sometimes me and my brothers had to wait till Nan came home or my auntie came up for us.

My younger brother always gets scared and he has to go to hospital with my mum. We all get scared.

Jasmine, 10

On Monday my Mum went into hospital. I had to stay at a friend's house for a while and I visited Mum on Friday and Saturday. I bought her some flowers and some chocolates, I had a lot of dreams and woke up crying. I was okay when I saw her. I started to feel happy.

On the Saturday I didn't find Mum in bed, that's when I started to worry but one of the nurses came and said, 'Are you looking for your Mum?' I didn't say anything. I was so upset when we found Mum, we caught her smoking in the garden. When I was telling her off I sounded like the mother. I was saying things like, 'Get back to bed. Do you want to kill yourself smoking? Give me your cigarette or put it out.'

In the morning I get up and if Mum's getting up I help her out of bed, if not I get ready for school and get her up when she's awake. When I arrive at school I'm fine until 11.00 am. Sometimes I'm okay and I just go to play but if I'm not I go to my head teacher and ask if I can phone my Mum. When I'm coming home I just go straight home unless my Mum asks me to go to the shop. When I get home I help do dinner if it needs doing and watch television, eat dinner, wash up, watch television some more and by 8.45 pm I get ready for bed, kiss Mum goodnight and I'm in bed by 9.00 pm. I read a book for 15 minutes and then it's another day in the morning.

M. (male), 16

Well me and dad are spectacular. What happened was, it all started off he got a slipped disc in his spine and he went in for an operation and they said he'd be fine. He's had the operation twice now. But the last time he had it he was paralysed, then he got moved to a physiotherapy unit, it was 24 hours physiotherapy and he's never been right since then.

He was told he was going to be all right after the first operation but it was just killing him 'cos he saw the shoulder and everything, and with him being right handed he couldn't write or anything, and he was getting worried. He went back and said something's gone wrong, do the operation again and it left him paralysed. He can't write, he can't sign things – I sign everything for him – and he finds it hard to walk a lot, so I do the shopping. He tends to stay in the house.

He's getting worse now. I tend to do everything really, basically he is a kid and I'm the father. I do the shopping, I clean the place, I make the beds, I do the washing, I do the cooking, I do all that. I'm a good cook.

I was only young, must have been about ten when it all started.

Sean, 12

I care for my brother and I get fed up
I really want to give him away but I cannot
I wish that people could understand how hard it is for me
I have a guilty feeling in my tummy

J. (female), 16

Mum had a massive hernia on her stomach. She was ill for three or four years. Just after she had [my brother] it blew up. She had an operation a year ago to remove it. Before that she was very very ill. She ended up getting septicaemia. So she was in hospital in and out going on two years. She couldn't go to the bathroom on her own, she couldn't walk. She couldn't go to bed – she just slept in the chair downstairs. So it was everything really. She couldn't cook, she couldn't clean, she couldn't look after my little brother. She was in a lot of pain, for a long time.

I used to go out maybe once a week with some friends. Just out on the street and stand on the streets. And I'd pop back every hour to see if [my brother] was all right and to see if she wanted anything. And then I'd come in and go to bed.

I left school before me sixteenth birthday. There was no phone calls, no letters, nothing. And I had my exams coming up that year as well which I'd been entered for. All they did was after the exams were done they sent me a bill. I'd been missing some school from when I was 12. They sent someone round and kept saying they were going to prosecute my mum for me not going to school. But it was actually more worry for her with her being ill as well. So I got registered with the Carers Association and they came and talked to me mum. And the social services said they couldn't actually prosecute me mum because I was caring for my mum.

If I'd have gone regularly to school I would have done all right. But under the circumstances I'd have felt I couldn't have gone. It would have just made me feel more guilty that I was going if you know what I mean. I just didn't want that.

My friends knew I was looking after my mum and that my mum was bad but that was it. I told one person. I'll never trust anybody ever again because she told the whole world about it. It was my business really. It was nobody else's. And eventually the school knew. A couple of the teachers were very nice to me really, they used to give me work to take home with me, and that used to help me a lot.

Social services came and they talked to my mum, and they mentioned to me mum about the Carers Association, and they came and talked to me about it and they asked if I wanted to meet them. And I said 'yeah', you know. That was two years ago. And I've recently sort of left it. I don't really have the time for it.

Rebecca, 15

My brother gets quite poorly
and sometimes so does my mum.
I help do some of the chores
I'm relieved when the day is done.
And the end of the day I get very tired and I just want to get into my bed,
I get onto the mattress and tightly pull the covers over my head.

I have to do a lot of work at school as well as work at home,
Home to me is very busy, at school I just roam.

I have to also have days off school to help my mum when she's ill,
I would pop down the chemist with her prescription to collect her pills.

There are many people in my house, we all take it in turn to help around,
As a little thank you I'd get money and I'd take my brother and sisters to the playground.

If I was to explain my typical day, my typical day would be:
waking up in the morning, do chores, have tea, go to bed and sleep.

Claire, 9

I look after my mum. She has a disease called Myasthenia Gravis. She can go into hospital any time when her muscles go weak. It affects her muscles, breathing, walking, speech etc. When my mum's ill I ring the ambulance. She tells me not to but I know it's for her own good!

When my mum's ill I go in a home with my sister. (My brother goes by his self.) When my mum comes out of hospital you can tell the difference but not for long. I help tidy up, undress her, help her in the bath, hoover, etc. After I've helped my mum there's a feeling inside of me which makes me happy.

My mum sees a lot of social workers and helpers. I get on with them fine, except one lady who takes me to school. At school most people understand especially my old year 3 teacher. If I get problems she helps me.

M. (male), 16

I have quite a few days off from school. Actually, since Christmas I haven't been to school. I went in and I said, 'I can't come in school because I need to help my dad', and they say, 'As long as you're in for your exams you're okay', which is fair enough. I used to miss at least a full week every month. I don't want to leave him – the school understand why – when I first joined the school I said, 'My dad's disabled so I'm going to have a lot of time off', and so they try and help as much as they can. What happens is I've got an agreement with the teachers if I ever feel worried or any thing then I can just walk out of school or the teachers will give me a lift home if I want one.

I joined this club for young carers, and the one who ran it was always going out for meals and she'd help me out – I talk to her all the time. It gets you out the house, talk to some people my age, 'cos there used to be eight of us, all different ages. Just used to go out and talk to each other, have a good laugh.

Margaret, 11

When I am working at school I am always worried about my Dad but when I am in the playground with my friends I just totally forget about him and have a good time.

When my Dad is having an operation I am always wondering if anything has happened to him.

Sometimes when I am running all around the house for him I get fed up with it.

When I am doing things for my Dad and my Tamagotchi is bleeping I just want to chuck it out of my bedroom window.

When I am cleaning up the house and my older brother wants me to do something for him I just want to magic him away 'cause he's getting on my nerves.

When my brother and sister are arguing they come running up to me and say nasty things about each other and I have enough to worry about, my Dad. I end up falling out with both of them, but in a way, when I think about it, I really like my brother and sister.

Sarah, 14

I have a twin sister and a younger sister who all have to care for our disabled Dad. He had a major stroke just over a year ago and is still very disabled from it. It has changed all of our lives a lot. It has affected our schoolwork, our relationship with our Dad and our daily lives. Instead of our Dad looking after us, it has changed and now we have to look after him. We have to cook, wash, clean and do most of the household jobs for both him and ourselves. When we want to go out with our friends, our Granny has to look after him. She has moved in now to help us but she is nearly 80 and can't manage everything that she would like to help out with.

J. (female), 18

If her arm was dead I used to have to help with the washing and
that. She always asked me to wash her hair because she couldn't
physically, even if her arm was good. It was hard for her to get her
head up so I'd always wash her hair for her and help her with it. If I
said, 'I don't want to do that mum' – like shaving under her arms – I
used to say, 'I don't want to do that mum'. She wouldn't make me
and if I said I didn't want do certain aspects of her bathing, she'd
say, 'Okay, I'll manage'. She always insisted for me and my brother
to be in the bathroom with her when she was having the bath –
whether she needed help or not – in the case of if she slipped down
or something and hit her head and that because she wasn't very
stable at times. She cannot – she will not – cook. She prefers not to,
not from the fact of laziness of cooking, because there was a time
she was cooking and she dropped a pan because it was too heavy
for her to lift.

Siobhan, 12

My mum has a back condition called spinal stenosis. This limits her
movements meaning she has to use walking sticks and aids around
the house. Also, mum needs a wheelchair whenever going further
than the garden.

This condition is hereditary, so maybe one day I will get it, or
maybe my 11 year old sister. Or maybe both of us.

Because of the way my mum is, I have had to grow up very quickly
– since I was six and my mum had a hysterectomy. I have to help a
lot around the house, although we have a lady that comes in to cook
our tea. Mum has always been so independent, and so it was hard
for her to have a stranger in the house to help when social services
found that I was cooking tea at nine years old.

I go to Young Carers, which relieves some of the pressure when I
know there are people who understand.

Melanie, 14

I can never predict which mood comes next.
Get her showered, dried and dressed.
Be the sister to meet her demands.
Cross the road and hold her hand.
Wipe her face after messy meals,
Try to understand the frustration she feels
When she's saying words that I can't make out,
And keep a clear head when she screams and shouts.
Stay interested in her persistent questions.
Help Mum and Dad and make suggestions.
Give them space, take her out for a walk,
Try to give them the time to talk.
Ignorant people quite often stare
At her expressive face and thinning hair,
She's someone different in their narrow view.
It makes me so angry, because if they knew
How much effect a child with learning difficulties has,
That a happy day with Katy erases ten that were bad.

C. (male), 16

He can't work. He lost his left side. So his left arm doesn't work,
and he can't walk on his left leg. I wash him, bath him, put him in
bed, dress him, go shopping, the little things like that. I'd just
turned 11 when [the stroke] happened. He can walk a bit with his
stick but he can't walk from there to here. He has to take his
wheelchair. He can't even move his hand at all. His hand is just
lodged there. It's very hard for him to dress. I do all the cooking. I
do all the shopping. Everything. For about five years now. I just got
used to it. I won't go nowhere until my dad, like, passes away.

R. (female), 13

What it's really like	What I wish
Lonely	Friends allowed home
No friends allowed home	Allowed to answer the phone and door
Not allowed to answer the phone or door	Can go and talk to family
Family always fall out	Can find it OK to go to school
Nowhere to turn	Not worried when I go out
Upsetting	Not to be tired all the time
Worrying	Not to lie anymore
Hard to go to school	To be a normal child
Tiring	Not to be treated like a 4 year old
Lying	
Treated like a 4 year old	

C. (male), 16

I empty her commode, do the kitchen, washing-up, most of the times I cook dinner… Collect her money from her social security, order her prescriptions, go down doctor's, get a prescription, then go down chemist – fetch tablets – bring them back, go down shop. Or if she's in the bath, just wash her hair or something when she can't do it herself. Stuff like that. Or at night time – because she has trouble getting out of a chair – so I have to lift her up and put her on the settee to go asleep, just stuff like that.

Mary-Jane, 13

… I used to care for my dad who is 66 and has got seven children ranging from 4–15 in age.

He is a good Dad considering he has got COAD [chronic obstructive airways disease] as well as asthma. But what topped it all off was when my youngest brother was only three months old my mum walked out on all seven of us, which was really difficult for me as I had to look after a three month old child and I was only ten and it just got too much for me looking after him, I mean I didn't have a clue what to do.

Over the next two years it was fine, then when I started my secondary school it was too much again. I was being bullied and then I had time off school to help around the house. The only person I could turn to was my niece.

But after a time my mum came back. Anyway things got more and more hard in 1999 because I had my Edinburgh Reading test. And in the Easter weeks I was being physically abused by my mum and what was worse is that it was for nothing. And on Easter Sunday I just walked out and didn't go back. I went to live with my sister and brother-in-law who has got rheumatoid arthritis, heart problems and cervical spondylitis. About two and a half years ago he had a double heart by-pass which has left him with angina. I try to help as much as possible around the home and that's all I can do.

Since I have been coming to Young Carers I have now been able to mingle with people and enjoy myself whereas before I didn't have a life.

Samantha, 14

When I was about ten years old my dad found out he had depression. My mum didn't tell me straight away because I was still quite young to understand. When I was told I was very scared because I didn't know anything about depression.

A couple of months went by after my mum had told me and I suddenly realised I was doing things I had never done before e.g. cooking, cleaning and paying bills. I also started falling behind with my schoolwork and getting into lots of trouble for falling asleep in class. My mum contacted the school and told them what I was going through. They were very understanding.

Helping out in the house doesn't bother me anymore. It is just like a routine now and it's good to help because then I know I am doing something for my dad, who I love very much. It does make me very tired at times but my mum always makes sure I get a rest. I also have a little sister and a big brother who help me and my mum very much.

G. (female), 17

A few friends did know but not many of them. My mum says, 'I'll tell the teachers why you've been away', and I went, 'No, no I don't want them to know', because you just feel like they take pity on you and everything and I said, 'No I don't want them to know', but mum says, 'That will explain your absences and then if you're not doing too good at school they'll know about it'. But when my mum went to a parents' evening the teachers were saying, 'No, no they're doing really good at school, they're all right'. So I says to mum, 'Don't say anything if they think we're doing all right at school, unless they say to you they're struggling', but I don't think mum ever told the teachers actually. I don't think I wanted my mum to tell the teachers at all. Friends knew but I think at one point my mum did ring one of the teachers because they were having problems with my younger sister and I think my mum ended up telling them what had happened but apart from that no one else knew really. It is only really my close friends.

Katie, 12

Dear Mum

I wish that you and me could spend some time together sometimes.

I feel really sad and left out.

You make me feel like a pair of hands, just there to help, instead of your daughter and although I am doing things that you tell me to I get really fed up.

We never have any personal time together because you never see me in the morning because you're asleep.

When I get home you send me to the shop or doctor's to fetch things and when I get back you go to sleep and I have to look after myself and my brothers and sisters. Then I make tea and when you wake up you send us to bed and it is like that every day and I really feel as though I am not there, **so please spend some time with me.**

J. (female), 16

I had to leave school in February because I was having a lot of time off to look after my mum. I weren't doing my homework and I missed out on a lot of coursework, which had to be in before my exams, so I never had enough coursework to be entered for all my exams, so I decided to leave. It wasn't worth it because I'd only been entered for two exams. So I left school to just look after my mum.

I've been doing it since nine. Housework, washing, washing-up, used to have to wash my mum as well. Just something I ended up doing. I do the decorating all through the house, front and back garden, cleaning the kitchen, everything, bedrooms, bathroom, all of it, I have to do it all. We used to have someone that used to come in to do the living room, but then you had to pay for it. We couldn't afford it to be paid for so we stopped it, and that's when I carried on doing it. But she needs someone to prepare her dinner, a meal, for the night-time. She can sometimes prepare a meal, but she can't dish it up. She can sit on a stool and peel some potatoes and some carrots, and that, but she can't hold a saucepan of anything because she drops it. So I do it normally. I learned. I'll still do the washing and my mum and dad's ironing, but it's absolutely everything, still.

She can get in and out the bath on her own, but you have to make sure she's okay. You have to keep popping up and down stairs. She couldn't be here on her own. I used to phone up from school but sometimes she couldn't hear the phone – if she was in the kitchen – and I used to get worried, and I used to walk out of school to come home to make sure she was all right. I was going in sometimes on a Tuesday, Wednesday, Thursday, Friday morning, or two times a week, or sometimes miss the whole week. It started from the second [secondary school] year. They used to think I used to make it up – as an excuse for not being in school. They sent a letter home, saying, 'Should not be missing school for any family problems whatsoever. Any school she does miss, she needs to catch up on', which is what I was doing. But because I was just copying it out of my friend's book it weren't going in the way it was going in with them, being explained to them. So what's the use in copying it all up if I ain't gonna understand what I'm writing? So, I gave up in the end.

Education welfare just say, 'It's no excuse for her to be off school, you need to get help in', but it's easier said than done. It's okay for them – they've got money, it's no problem. But having the money problems that we had, it's quite expensive now to have a carer in. But I just used to ignore them. I couldn't go, mum was more important. The Education person came in the January this year, saying that if I wasn't in school my mum and my dad would be took to court. But it takes just over six months to get it processed through a court, so by that time I would've been on exam leave anyway. So I haven't bothered and no one's said anything since.

If my mum never had the stroke I'd probably still be in school. All my coursework would have been in, everything. I would have been able to concentrate on just one thing – on school – and then, perhaps, I would have gone to college. Perhaps I would have just gone straight into work, I'll never know now. I mean, perhaps I might be where I am now, I might have left school, you know, but I probably would have stayed on at school to do my GCSEs, do what grades I could have done, and then gone on to work. Going to work, earning your own little bit of income, I would probably have been more like that than what I am now.

Abigale, 11

Read this to all teachers.

Some people can't get their homework done because they are under lots of pressure and stress, so don't say they are lazy because you don't understand.

You should listen to them.

Instead of saying they're lazy you should give them their word so just let them say what they want to say and don't Butt In!!

PLEASE LISTEN!!!!!!!!!

You have to go to school to learn and some people might think you have to have a break.

That is why you go to school.

When you go to school it makes me mad when people make fun of the disabled people and when it comes to homework.

You say why you have not done your work and you tell them what you have done.

They say You Told Me That Last Week. You Are Lying To Me.

Lucie, 15

My mum has a bad back and has battled against cancer three times and she has had to have a nerve removed from her leg. She has had to go into hospital for operations on her back. Because my dad works away from home, when my mum goes into hospital me and my brother have to have a home help/carer to come in and look after us.

When my dad is away I have to look after my mum and younger brother. I have to cook, clean the house and help my mum. I have to fetch my mum's pills and help her to get out of bed. It's hard work and sometimes I feel really tired. This is made worse because I have to go out to work to earn my pocket money etc. It makes me feel happy though when my mum says thank you.

My teachers don't really understand what I have to do at home. My mum does not like people to know how ill she is, it's really hard for her to tell them. I have to have a lot of time off school to care for my mum because I can't leave her on her own. Because of this I have now been put on an alternative programme at school, which means I can finish at lunch times.

When my dad is away, I become responsible for everybody and the house.

I don't get on with social workers because they keep trying to take me and my brother away from my mum when my dad is working.

I am involved in a young carers group which meets every Wednesday night. This means I can get out of the house and have a laugh with my friends. The group gives you the support you need and a chance to meet other carers, we also go on trips out and camping trips.

As I get older I have to take on more responsibility and it gets harder for me.

Rah, 13

I think social workers are stupid because I had my first one when I was about seven. They didn't come round to see me! I never saw them! The next thing I knew I was in a strange house with total strangers.

My Mum went frequently into hospital since then, me and my brother went to stay with close friends. Again I never saw them (social workers). I lost trust in them and felt alone.

We then moved house and I think social services just forgot about me and my brothers. I didn't see them for about two years. We then had to move up to [name of town]. We lived in a strange place. She went into hospital again. Caroline came round to speak to me and I started coming to Share the Care. My Mum went in hospital soon after. I met my social worker at the hospital. He said he would come and see me next week. I didn't see him for about two months. My Mum rang up and explained what happened. They said they would sort it out and said they would see us next week. They didn't come. My Mum ended up going to their offices, but of course they said the same thing again.

Now I never see them. My social worker has now left! So now they should know what is happening.

SO PLEASE TAKE NOTICE!

D. (female), 18

I would always go shopping for food and I used to cook. When my brothers used to come I used to cook for them. In the morning my mum used to do breakfasts and everything when she was sober. But when it got towards the day, through the day till evening she used to get drunk more, she used to drink more and more. I used to cook food when they used to come and for my mum every other day. If I didn't cook for myself I would have just starved.

When I used to go to school sometimes she used to try and bribe me, because she did get lonely. She didn't like to stay in the house on her own. When I used to go out to school she used to say, 'I'll give you some money if you stay off school', and I used to say 'no' because I liked school. If I wanted to stay at my dad's house at the weekends she used to get upset and say that she didn't want to be left alone. If I ever wanted to stay at a friend's house she used to get really angry because I was leaving her and she didn't want to be by herself.

About 50 per cent of school I missed because of staying at home looking after my mum. When she was in hospital I had time off going to see her. After the first year I spoke to my form tutor who asked me about it and I told her about her drink problem. The head of the year as well. I explained to her why my attendance was bad. They understood but they tried to encourage me to come to school. I mean I like school but it still didn't stop me worrying when I went to school. When I did exams, I did quite well. Weller than what I expected with my GCSEs because I expected to get nothing.

I was surprised that the social workers didn't do anything, you know. Even talk about me being put into foster care. When we were living with my mum and I were really looking after her and she was drinking a lot and threatening to take her own life, they came up to visit sometimes to see how she were, but they never ever mentioned even thinking about putting me into foster care. They didn't say, 'Oh you're in danger' or anything. If they had wanted me to go in I don't think I would have because I would have wanted to stay with my mum. Because I would have been worried.

S. (female), 17

When you're younger you don't really understand what's happening. You know this person as your mum and you think, oh yeah I really love my mum. Then suddenly they turn into a totally different person and you can't understand. You're trying to relate what they're doing to the person that you've known all your life and you can't do it, and you get really confused.

I've started gradually being more understanding about what my mum does when she's ill. Last year she was really bad. She used to cry, she'd sit in a dark room and just cry and cry and I'd try and help her and when I used to say something to her she used to swear at me and tell me to get lost and I couldn't do anything and she'd just be crying. I could hear her upstairs and I didn't know what to do and then she'd just say really weird things as well, and I just had to keep telling myself that it wasn't her – if you know what I mean – it was her but I kept having to say, 'Well this is the illness that's speaking, not herself', and it's really hard. It's really confusing because there's somebody saying really weird things and you can't relate to what they're saying and you're trying to communicate with them and you can't because you can't understand them and you're not on their level and it's really, really confusing.

You don't get any sympathy from anybody either because when you try to explain to your friends – say your friend will ring up and your mum will answer the phone and she'll be saying really weird things to them and then you'll get back to school and everybody will start picking on you saying, 'Oh your mum's a nutter, she's a schizophrenic' – and that's a totally different illness anyway. And people never understand because a lot of people are really ignorant. You never get any of the support you would if your mum had got a physical illness because a lot of people, if your mum had cancer or something, they'd feel really sorry for you, but when's it's a mental illness people react so differently and they just like slag you to the ground saying, 'Oh your mum's a total nutter, she's a fruitcake', and it really upsets me. So, apart from having to deal with that you're having to deal with everybody else's reactions as well and it's just really hard trying to explain to people. I mean my mum's not a nutter, she's just really depressed, she doesn't go out doing really silly things and stabbing people and talking to the television, she just gets really depressed and she talks to herself. I think that's because she hasn't got anybody else to talk to really so she talks to herself. It's just her way of channelling her anger and her bitterness out of what's happened in the past, but a lot of people won't try to understand and then I lose my temper sometimes when people are just so ignorant.

When she's ill she stops washing and everything so I was like washing the clothes. I know it's not much really, just washing the clothes and I didn't really mind … and like cooking and stuff, 'cause my mum just lets herself go, she doesn't even clean herself, she just loses … doesn't see herself as important and she just doesn't do anything. But I don't think that's very hard really, doing that, I mean I don't mind. It's when you're having to deal with all the psychological aspects of it, when you're having to sort of understand … and it's really hard, you know, when people say really strange things and you can't even try to understand it.

You don't fully sleep when she's up. You're always getting up and going into her bedroom to see if she's all right. Once she was really crying and she was talking into the mirror to herself and my sister's father – he's dead now because he took a drug overdose and he was a really depressed man – and she would talk to the mirror, into the mirror at him, saying, 'Are you there?', and that was really weird as well and I kept having to get up in the middle of the night to see that she hadn't done anything to herself.

J. (female), 17

I was probably about 12 or 13 I think, not any far back than that really because that's when it really started being noticeable. I mean I knew he was, always knew he was taking medication but when you're young you don't really seem to ask questions. You just think he might have something wrong with him but when he started drinking and getting abusive towards my mum and that and he was drinking a lot more and he told me he wasn't taking the drugs any more because they made him worse and things, that's when I started recognising there was something more than, like, a cut leg. It was more inside the head and that. So then I started questioning my mum and she told me a lot more. Then I started getting a lot nosier about work because he kept coming home stressed from work and every time he came home from work he used to argue with my mum so I knew there was something wrong with the job. And then she went on about his job and then she eventually told us about the actual illness itself, and just went through things like the arguments, the shouting, hitting, things like that. And then he started shouting at me because I used to stick up for my mum and things so, yeah, I was about 12, 13 when I started, you know.

He's been in hospital a few times. He didn't go in willingly – they had to section him. At that point I used to say to mum, 'Well why won't he go in, if the doctors say he's poorly why won't he go in?' So then she used to say to me, 'Well, because he's got a mental illness and he doesn't understand', and then she used to tell me more and then he obviously got sectioned and then the police actually arrested him a few times in front of us three because he was carrying on and sectioned him personally, that's when my mum told us more as well because I didn't understand why, you know, how they could just put someone in hospital. I thought they had to have their consent etc. and then my mum started telling us a lot more about it saying he's got a mental illness, he's got to go in there, best place for him. Then we actually visited him and it was an awful experience. He used to just say, 'Oh them dickheads have put me in here, it's these drugs they're giving me, that's what sent me like I am.' That's why I needed to know more because I thought, 'My dad – what's he on about? It's his fault he's in there', and I never really knew whose fault it was, you can't blame anyone so that's why I wanted to know more about it so a lot of the information came from my mum really because I didn't really want to talk about it with anyone else because my mum had experienced it all her life.

It was just difficult for us you know because when you go to school everyone is happy and you're upset. And when we did go to school people was like saying, 'Why have you been off?' and it was like, 'My dad's been poorly', 'But why?' and like I couldn't say to them, 'He's got a mental illness', because half of them wouldn't even understand, you know, like they'd call him 'schizo', you know, 'psycho', something like that. That really upsets me that so I never told anybody really, so I just said I'd been ill or my Gran was poorly. I'd just make up anything really but the teacher knew why but obviously the students didn't. That was based over about two years, it wasn't like four months off school but it still meant a lot because it was catch-up time so we missed a lot of work really.

Now I've seen my dad being depressed it's like when I get so depressed I think, 'I'd better not start having it'. I mean I don't think I will but there's always the thing in the back of your mind. I mean I see myself sometimes as depressed like my dad and I sometimes think, you know, 'God I'd better not be turning out like my dad with an illness like that', but my mum always reassures me it's just my way of handling things really, touch wood.

S. (female), 17

Mum's got osteo- and that other arthritis. She's got both. Mainly in her hips and legs. She's had two hip replacements, but she's got it in her knees and stuff and sometimes in her hands. She can walk, but not very far, round the house she's okay. When she goes to church, she's okay, but if I actually wanted to go to the shops or anything, we have to take her in a wheelchair.

I do most of the evening things, like cooking meals, cleaning round the house and make sure everything's tidy, because she's quite house-proud, and that makes it really hard for her really. Being house-proud everything has to be in a certain place. Because she can't do it all the time I have to make sure that it's like that, otherwise she gets stressed out. So I have to make sure that everything is okay and I clean and tidy, and cook. Mum manages to put the washing actually in the washer, but I have to bring it down from upstairs, and then take the drying and the ironing and stuff back upstairs. We get a lady in from home help to do our ironing, she comes for an hour, so whatever she gets done in that hour is done, and if she doesn't, then I have to do the rest.

She needs emotional support, a lot. She gets very upset because the fact that she can't go out, and she sees all her friends, or other people going out. They come and visit her – that's great – but they go out like other places, and they go on holiday, and it really upsets her that she can't.

A lot of people would probably feel sorry for me. I don't want them to, because, you know, it's my mum that I'm looking after. That's sort of like one of my duties, and you know, because I love her that much, that's what I'm doing it for. Some people are like, 'Oh, you look after your mum, you're so good', and it's like 'yeah', but it's not like that. I do it because I love her, and not because I want any praise or any sympathy or anything like that.

Julie, 16

I don't think anyone would choose to be a 'carer' at any age, and while you are young it can be especially difficult. But I know that it is this that has made me who I am and has changed my life in many ways. All this despite the temporary difficulties. I like to see things in a positive light and would like any young carers who may read this to think positively too.

At times being a carer is tiring and soul-destroying. I battle against an invisible disease in my brother that means his health deteriorates, but the signs are very visible and as a family we must deal with them. I am the only one who can give him emotional support when he is feeling down. Our parents drive him round the bend (surprise surprise!) and it's me who's left to make him smile when he's going through hard times. It's me who is there to make him laugh when there's absolutely nothing to laugh about. However much hard work it is to achieve this, it's always worthwhile for the smiles and look he gives me. However much I 'give' to him, the amount he 'gives' back in return far exceeds this.

The time I spend with my brother is based around making sure he has the time of his life now, because he may not later. I could live five times longer than him, so his quality of life is important to me. It's great when we go out somewhere excellent, or go on holiday, because he enjoys it even if it's not 'my idea of fun'.

Being a young carer teaches you so much, perhaps taking away childhood, but often giving you an awareness of life and how precious it is. Some would say I've had to grow up too fast, but I believe I've made more of my life because of it.

Sometimes I feel like I have to make up for what he can't do. I try to be two children in one. I did this in my GCSE's and do it in my hobbies, in my social life too. But it all boils down to the fact that I don't want to waste any opportunity I have got because I've seen just what it's like to have none at all.

Some people do the things they want to because they choose to. Young carers don't always get the choice, but what we want is not sympathy and apologies for our supposed misfortune, but recognition and encouragement for what we do.

Good Practice Checklists

The rights of young carers

All family members have rights. Each young carer is both a child or young person, *and* a carer, and has rights as such under legislation: the Children Act, the Carers (Recognition and Services) Act and the UN Convention on the Rights of the Child. Young carers have …

- the right to self-determination and choice (to be children, carers or both)
- the right to be recognised and treated separately from the care receiver
- the right to be heard, listened to and believed
- the right to privacy and respect
- the right to play, recreation and leisure
- the right to education
- the right to health and social care services specific to their needs
- the right to practical help and support, including respite care
- the right to protection from physical and psychological harm (including the right to protection from injury caused by lifting etc.)
- the right to be consulted and be fully involved in discussions about decisions which affect their lives and the lives of their families
- the right to information and advice on matters that concern them and their families (including benefits and services, medical information etc.)
- the right to access to trained individuals and agencies who can deliver information and advice with appropriate expertise, in confidence
- the right to independent and confidential representation and advocacy, including befriending or 'buddying'
- the right to a full assessment of their needs, strengths and weaknesses, including full recognition of racial, cultural and religious needs
- the right to appeal and complaints procedures that work
- the right to stop physically caring.

Source: J. Aldridge and S. Becker, *Children who Care* (Young Carers Research Group, 1993), pp. 78–9.

Checklist for GPs and health professionals

Finding out the facts

- Check whether parents with disabilities or long-term illness are receiving any support, assistance or care in the home, and if so who provides it. You may find that a child is providing care, either alone or with another adult. Children are more likely to act as carers if the ill person is a lone parent, but even in two-parent families children may take on significant caring responsibilities.

- Make links between patients, particularly ill or disabled parents, and their families, so that you can assess how the health or disability of a parent might impact on a child, or vice versa. For example, including an up to date family tree in health records can assist in the identification of who provides care in the family.

- Where children are seeking medical attention because of strained backs, or have emotional or behavioural problems, check whether this may be linked in any way with the illness or disability of a family member, particularly a parent. The presenting symptom may be caused by the child having to take on inappropriate caring responsibilities in the home.

- If you have reason to believe (from speaking with a parent or child) that children may be providing care for parents or other family members, find out *what* it is that they are having to do, and *why* they are having to do it.

Working with other agencies

- If you have established that children are providing substantial, regular or significant care to another family member, then speak to parents and children about this, either separately or together, and ask whether they need help and support to prevent children from having to continue to provide care, or to reduce their responsibilities.

- Young carers have a right to an assessment of their needs from social services, but many do not know about this. Talk to them about their rights, and help them access social services if this is what they want.

- Be prepared to make a referral to another agency for specialist support or services. The local social services department should assess the ill or disabled person, and they should assess the child, as a carer under the Carers Act or perhaps as a child in need under the Children Act. There may also be a local young carers project which can provide activities, counselling and other support to the young carer.

Further reading: S. Becker, C. Dearden and J. Aldridge, 'Young carers', in L. Polnay (ed.), *Community Paediatrics* (Harcourt Brace, 2000).

Checklist for teachers and school staff

Finding out the facts

- Where children regularly miss school, or are late, seem tired in class, are underachieving, have behavioural problems or are failing to do homework, always check whether this is linked in any way with the long-term illness or disability of a family member, particularly a parent. The child's problems may be caused by having to take on inappropriate caring responsibilities in the home. Children and young people are more likely to become carers if they live in a one-parent family which does not receive adequate professional support or services, *and* is living on a low income.

- If you have reason to believe that children may be providing care for parents or other family members, find out *what* it is that they are having to do, and *why* they are having to do it.

- Once you have established that children are providing substantial, regular or significant care to another family member, speak to parents and children about this, either separately or together, and ask whether they are receiving the help and support they need to help children to reduce their responsibilities, *and* to ensure that they can make the most of their schooling.

Working with other agencies

- Children and young people who act as carers have a right to an assessment of their needs from social services, but many do not know about this. Talk to them about their rights, and help them access social services if this is what they want.

- Be prepared to make a referral to another agency for specialist support or services, again if this is what children and parents want. The local social services department should assess the ill or disabled person and also the child, either as a carer under the Carers Act or as a child in need under the Children Act. There may also be a local young carers project which can provide activities, counselling and other support to the young carer.

- Each school should have a designated person who keeps up to date with the research and policy on young carers, and who can be used as a resource by other teachers for advice and information. They should know about any local projects and people in other agencies (health, education welfare service, social services etc.) who have particular expertise.

How the school can help

- It is necessary to strike a sensible balance between collusion ('it's all right to miss school if you are caring') and punitive intervention (the threat of court proceedings if children don't attend school).

- Schools can compound educational difficulties by failing to recognise young carers' specific needs and by not entering them for examinations. Every effort should be made to help young carers who are having problems at school achieve the educational qualifications they will need for adult life and future employment.

- Schools should develop resources – for example a club, special group or one-to-one teaching – to give young carers who have missed school learning opportunities to enable them to cover coursework. Home tuition may be required, but it is generally better for children to be educated at school with their contemporaries.

- Many young carers say they are bullied at school because a member of their family is disabled and they are having to provide care for him or her. It may be appropriate to introduce in assembly or classroom some sessions on disability awareness, to break down negative images, stereotypes and prejudices.

- Children may want to keep their family circumstances strictly private; their wishes must be respected.

Further reading: C. Dearden and S. Becker, *Growing Up Caring* (National Youth Agency, 2000).

Checklist for social workers

Finding out the facts

- Find out whether parents with disabilities or long-term illness are receiving any support, assistance or care in the home, and if so who provides it. You may find that a child is providing care, either alone or with another adult. Children and young people are more likely to become carers if they live in a one-parent family which does not receive adequate professional support or services, *and* is living on a low income.

- Where children have health or social problems, such as a strained back, or emotional, behavioural or educational difficulties (e.g. they miss school, are often late, are tired in class, underachieve or are failing to do homework), always check whether this might be linked in any way with having to care for another family member, particularly a parent.

- If, from speaking with a parent or child, you have reason to believe that children may be providing care for parents or other family members, find out *what* it is that they are having to do, and *why* they are having to do it.

Making an assessment

- If you have established that children are providing substantial, regular or significant care to another family member, then speak to parents and children about this, either separately or together, and ask what help and support they each need to prevent children from having to continue to provide care, or to reduce their responsibilities. You may want to think about using a Family Group Conference approach to these discussions.

- Young carers have a right to an assessment of their needs from social services, but many families do not know about this. Talk to them about their rights to an assessment as a carer under the Carers Act or as a child in need under the Children Act, and help them access this assessment if that is what they want. (There is a separate checklist on assessments on page 78.) Assessments must recognise the needs and rights of all family members and services must be responsive to the needs of young carers *and* disabled parents.

The whole family

- Interventions must focus on the needs of the whole family. Those which support ill or disabled parents, including offering help with parenting, will provide the best way forward. Services should be developed which cater for the needs of disabled parents and young carers.

- The emphasis must be on preventing children from taking on inappropriate caring roles in the first place, and stopping these roles from becoming firmly established once started.

Working with other agencies

- Be prepared to make a referral to another agency for specialist support or services. There may also be a local young carers project which can provide activities, counselling and other support to the young carer.

- Each social services department should have a designated person who keeps up to date with the research and policy on young carers, and who can be used as a resource by other social workers for advice and information. They should know about any local projects and people in other agencies (health, education, the voluntary sector etc.) who have particular expertise.

Further reading: S. Becker, J. Aldridge and C. Dearden, *Young Carers and their Families* (Blackwell Science, 1998).

Do's and don'ts when assessing young carers

- **Do** arrange the assessment in advance, with both the child and the parent(s).
- **Do** ask the young carer, in private, whether they would like their parent(s) to be present during assessment.
- **Do** ask the young carer whether they would like to be assessed at home or elsewhere.
- **Do** explain fully, in age-appropriate language, what assessment is about and why they are being assessed.
- **Do** listen to what carers have to say and acknowledge their preferences.
- **Do** allow enough time for a full assessment – one visit will often be insufficient.
- **Do** encourage the young carer to have an advocate present if desired (and explain clearly what an advocate is and why they may be useful).
- **Do** give children written feedback, in age-appropriate language, of the outcomes of their assessment and discuss this with them in person to ensure they understand what services or support are to be offered (or why they cannot be provided at this time).

- **Don't** make value-laden assumptions with regard to gender, age, ethnicity etc.
- **Don't** use jargon.
- **Don't** assume that children will understand the term 'assessment' in the same way adults do – for children it is often associated with school exams and tests.
- **Don't** provide time-limited services without ensuring that the young carer is aware that they *are* time-limited and will be withdrawn at a later date.

Source: C. Dearden and S. Becker, *Young Carers in the UK: A Profile* (Carers National Association, 1998), p. 79.

References and
Further Reading

J. Aldridge and S. Becker, *Children who Care: Inside the World of Young Carers* (Young Carers Research Group, Loughborough University, 1993).

J. Aldridge and S. Becker, *My Child, My Carer: The Parents' Perspective* (Young Carers Research Group, Loughborough University, 1994).

J. Aldridge and S. Becker, *Befriending Young Carers: A Pilot Study* (Young Carers Research Group, Loughborough University, 1996).

J. Aldridge and S. Becker, *The National Handbook of Young Carers Projects*, 1998 edition (Carers National Association in association with Young Carers Research Group, Loughborough University, 1998).

S. Becker, J. Aldridge and C. Dearden, *Young Carers and their Families* (Blackwell Science, 1998).

S. Becker and R. Silburn, *We're in This Together: Conversations with Families in Caring Relationships* (Carers National Association, 1999).

S. Becker, 'Carers', *Research Matters*, October 1999–April 2000.

S. Becker, C. Dearden and J. Aldridge, 'Young carers', in L. Polnay (ed.) *Community Paediatrics* (Harcourt Brace, 2000).

H. Crabtree and L. Warner, *Too Much to Take On: A Report on Young Carers and Bullying* (The Princess Royal Trust for Carers, 1999).

M. Crawford, 'Choices for families', *Journal of Young Carers Work*, October 1999.

D. Deacon, 'Young carers and old hacks', *Journal of Young Carers Work*, April 1999.

C. Dearden, S. Becker and J. Aldridge, *Partners in Caring: A Briefing for Professionals about Young Carers* (Young Carers Research Group, Carers National Association, Crossroads UK, 1994).

C. Dearden and S. Becker, *Young Carers – The Facts* (Community Care magazine, 1995).

C. Dearden and S. Becker, *Young Carers in the UK: A Profile* (Carers National Association, 1998).

C. Dearden and S. Becker, *Growing Up Caring: Vulnerability and Transition to Adulthood – Young Carers' Experiences* (National Youth Agency, 2000).

C. Dearden and S. Becker, 'Young carers: needs, rights and assessments', in J. Howarth (ed.), *The Child's World: The Reader* (Stationery Office, 2000).

Department of Health, *Caring about Carers: A National Strategy for Carers* (Department of Health, 1999).

J. Frank, C. Tatum and S. Tucker, *On Small Shoulders* (The Children's Society, 1999).

S. Hill, 'The physical effects of caring on children', *Journal of Young Carers Work*, October 1999.

R. Howell, 'When is a project not a project?', *Journal of Young Carers Work*, October 1998.

The Independent, 'Children who care: their stories are different', *The Independent*, 3 September 1998.

Joint Consultative Committee (Liverpool), *Young Carers' Mental Health Resource Pack* (City of Liverpool, 1999).

Journal of Young Carers Work, 'Caring and coping: a story of mental illness' (interview with Dr Lynne Jones MP), *Journal of Young Carers Work*, April 1998.

L. Keith and J. Morris, 'Easy targets: a disability rights perspective on the "children as carers" debate', *Critical Social Policy*, 44/45, pp. 36–57.

R. Olsen, 'Young carers and the "disability" response: identifying common ground', *Journal of Young Carers Work*, April 1999.

L. Shore, 'The language of coping and caring', *Journal of Young Carers Work*, October 1999.

Young Carers Research Group website. Up-to-date information on young carers research, reports, and projects in the UK, and an annotated bibliography of all publications on young carers, including all YCRG publications can be found on: www.lboro.ac.uk/departments/ss/centres/YCRG/ycrg.htm